Ketogenic Diet

The complete guide to a high-fat diet, free recipes for busy people on the Keto diet, easy meal plans heal your body, and regain your self-confidence

"Your Essential Guide to Keto"

By "Wiley Pearson"

©2018

KETOGENIC DIET

The complete guide to a high-fat diet, free recipes for busy people on the Keto diet, easy meal plans heal your body, and regain your self-confidence

"Your Essential Guide to Keto"

By "Wiley Pearson"

Introduction

Hi everyone, before we begin I have some inquiry for you,

- ✓ Are you overweight?
- ✓ Are you hunting down sound life?
- ✓ Can't wear your most loved garments?
- ✓ Feel bashful when you are with companions?
- ✓ Always feel tired, or out of energy?
- ✓ Have some medical issues due to over weight?
- ✓ Tried numerous diet regimens with no outcome?

On the off chance that your answer is **"yes"** for at least one of these inquiries, so you are in the correct place and opportune time to change your life for eternity.

Numerous inquiries we are spend our life's in scanning for their answers!!! A few of us found however greater part are as yet looking and seeking.

These days you will discover hundreds might be even a huge number of books, Magazines, TV appears, and so forth.... discussing similar subjects, they give us great information yet the vast majority of us can't take after because of our way of life.

In this book you will locate a full manual for begin your new existence with the Ketogenic Diet System which you can take after effortlessly with no endure.

Shall we get started?

Why I wrote this book?

I wrote this book as I want you to escape the Dieting Trap and Transform Your Life

Have you been spinning your wheels, trying diet after diet, only to lose and regain the same 10, 20, or 30 pounds over and over again? Author Ari Whitten's here to tell you that it's not your fault! The common weight loss strategy of "burn more calories than you take in" will fail 95% of you in the long term, simply because this goes against your body's natural wisdom. So it's time to stop fighting against your biology and start working with your biology. Forever Fat Loss will show you how.

Why you should read this book?

Do you sense that you haven't been honored with the best fat consuming hereditary qualities? Does sustenance appear to go straight to your concern territories like your paunch, bum and thighs?

Do you sense that you've attempted each diet known to man however the weight continues returning?

Imagine a scenario in which I revealed to you that you could get thinner, can rest easy, look better, have more energy, decrease torment, help your sex drive, anticipate infection ... and best of all despite everything you'll have the capacity to in any case eat a portion of the sustenance you desire the most and still experience a slimmer body.

In Ketogenic Diet that is precisely what you'll get

You will find the correct science behind how we put on and get in shape and in addition what completely should be done to assault that tenacious muscle versus fat; that as of recently has been so testing to dispose of. The procedures in this book are so basic, so natural to actualize thus effective... That it will presumably stable so mind boggling when you first read about it.

This weight pulverizing day by day propensities will convey you an aggregate body changeover with no supplements, sweat-soaked exercises or overrated ineffectual weight reduction pills. It will deal with individuals of any weight, anyone shape and anyone write.

Is this book for you?

Way of life isn't a prevailing fashion diet. Comprehend brain science and realize why being overweight isn't your blame.

Getting in shape is similarly as simple as ever on the off chance that you will change some of your day by day propensities, so it is your choice

In this book we will discover how to improve life by simply following a simple and all around composed framework for your life

About The Author

I'm able to sense your-suffer as I was simply for your place long term in the past, I used to be over weigh, fat, hiding my body with heavy clothes even in summer time!!!

However now I'm totally exclusive, yes consider me when I say you and only you most effective can determine what precisely you need to looks as if.

Start nowadays and that I'm a 100% sure that you'll reach your dream.

I'm a normal man, having normal life, married with one child and I'm scripting this book due to the fact I need to help human beings as I got assist from near friend that point which surely modified my life.

Want you all the pleasant,

The author

Table of content

Sweet snacks

Conclusion

Author Final words

One last thing

If you enjoyed this book or find it useful, I'd be very grateful if you would post short review on Amazon, your support really does make a difference and I read all of the reviews personally so I can get your feedback and make that book even better.

If you would like to give a review, then all you need to do is click the reviewer link on this book's page on Amazon here

Thanks again for your support.

Let's Get Started!!!

Ketogenic Diet life style,

Introduction:

The Ketogenic diet is a high-fat, moderate-protein, low-carbohydrate diet that was utilized before to treat epilepsy in children who did not recuperate well to the accessible epilepsy medicines around then.

This diet style upholds the body to utilize and consume fats as the fundamental wellspring of energy over than utilizing carbohydrates. The body changes the taken carbohydrates in our nourishment into glucose which later is sent all through the body to be used as energy. Shockingly, if your carbohydrates intake is higher than your body needs for the amount of energy you use during a day, the overabundance glucose is changed over fats and stored rather than being burned causing weight gain.

Be that as it may, in the event that you confine the measure of carbohydrates ingested, the liver will start changing over fat into unsaturated fats and ketone bodies. When ketones in the blood dwarf the molecules of glucose, the cells of your body will begin to utilize those ketones as their fundamental wellspring of energy.

How Does The Ketogenic Diet Work?

The Ketogenic diet fills in as it moves the body's metabolism from utilizing glucose as energy to utilize ketones to be the principle wellspring of energy. While it doesn't ensure moment weight reduction, it is a compelling diet framework to help you to accomplish your objectives of living in healthier way and make the most of your life.

In the first place, you will be eating extremely fulfilling and nutritious nourishments that will influence you to encounter fewer desires and to be less eager frequently. The present nutritionists won't disclose to you that great fats cause satiation, not foods grown from the ground. It has been resolved through numerous restorative examinations that protein and fats are the most fulfilling of the three macronutrients you will be worried about when following this new way of life.

Second, eating fats really encourages your body to consume the put away fat with the goal that you can shed pounds in a less demanding way.

Carbohydrates make the body create insulin to move glucose particles into the cells to be utilized for energy. Sadly, almost everybody who is overweight for a drawn out stretch of time will encounter some type of insulin-resistance regardless of whether they have not been analyzed as diabetic.

This implies you will encounter both high and low glucose levels and also more yearnings.

Also, third, you will have the capacity to accomplish more prominent weight loss because of the metabolic preferred standpoint the low-carbohydrates diet underpins.

At the point when your liver separate fats there are constantly a greater number of ketones than your body can really utilize, so the overabundance is discharged through pee

In any case, that loss of potential energy isn't excessively extraordinary so you won't miss it.

Comparison between Ketogenic Diet and 'Traditional' Diets

You may have attempted maybe a couple – or many – of the more traditional diets and had a long time to a couple of months worth of weight reduction yet thought that it was anything but difficult to ... suppose, fudge your diet? Furthermore, I imply that actually – fudge can be a major destruction. Am I right?

Presently we can Compare the accompanying two records and perceive how the Ketogenic diet can help you to accomplish your weight loss objectives.

Traditional Diet

- ✓ Restricts fat admission

- ✓ Allows for direct protein admission

- ✓ Increases leafy foods consumption (fruits and vegetables)

- ✓ Follows Food Pyramid rules

- ✓ Restricts caloric admission

- ✓ Doesn't enable changes in accordance with decrease abundance hunger

- ✓ Doesn't mitigate longings

- ✓ May require obtaining extraordinarily bundled dinners relying upon what diet is being taken after

Ketogenic Diet

- ✓ Restricts carbohydrates consumption

- ✓ Allows for direct protein consumption

- ✓ Increases advantageous fat admission

- ✓ Flips the Food Pyramid rules on its head

- ✓ Restricting caloric admission isn't completely vital

- ✓ Allows change in accordance with decrease abundance hunger

✓ Alleviates most, if not all, desires

✓ Doesn't require uniquely bought sustenance unless you do as such

As should be obvious, the Ketogenic diet is the inverse of any traditional diet you may have attempted. Perhaps that is the reason it works so well.

Ketogenic Diet is Dangerous!!

How frequently did you hear that the Ketogenic diet is unsafe to your wellbeing? Some, right!!

Indeed, even specialists have been known to state this same thing. In any case, these 'perils' are only myths passed on by individuals who have a constrained comprehension of low carb diets and how they function.

One of the principle reactions is that since it's a high fat diet that it will make you have a higher shot of heart related issues. The message that fat is the thing that influences you to fat has been drummed into the aggregate cognizance of Americans throughout the previous 30 years or more. This message has been rehashed again and again however it is a lie.

It's exceptionally hard to unlearn a lie that you've been instructed for most, if not all, of your life. Actually a high carb-diet drives up your glucose and insulin levels.

Sugar and insulin causes irritation in your body. The fats permitted on the Ketogenic diet are soaked fats and keeping in mind that immersed fats are sound for you, when joined in the standard American diet it gets the fault for causing coronary illness. This is on the grounds that it was examined in mix with a high starch diet.

The Ketogenic diet, which is high in soaked fat and low in carbohydrates, will really diminish irritation as a result of the lessening of glucose and insulin levels in your body.

Another feedback is that high admission of immersed fats and cholesterol causes coronary diseases. This is another lie that has been sustained for numerous decades. Another examination from understand American Medical School says that the Ketogenic diet is more beneficial in light of the higher soaked fat admission. Higher immersed fat admission expands HDL (great) cholesterol.

In the meantime, the lower sugar consumption diminishes triglyceride levels. These are the two factors that are the markers for coronary illness; the nearer your triglyceride and HDL levels are to 1, the more beneficial your heart. It is realized that coronary illness is caused by expending an abnormal state of carbohydrates consistently as opposed to high soaked fat utilization.

A third feedback is that individuals don't do well in ketosis. This isn't totally valid. As will be talked about later in this book, you ought to counsel with your doctor before beginning a Ketogenic diet program and in the event that you have certain previous medicinal conditions then you ought to either maintain a strategic distance from the way of life or be entirely administered by your restorative care supplier.

In any case, it has been discovered that our Stone Age man progenitors made due in a condition of consistent ketosis since grains were extremely hard to accumulate in substantial amounts and the grains they gathered were not as much handled as the carbohydrates expended today.

However another feedback "conceivably the most damning yet to the least extent liable to happen" is that there is the threat of a man following the Ketogenic diet to fall into Ketoacidosis.

Ketoacidosis is a perilous condition however basically being in ketosis isn't sufficient to make you build up this condition.

Ketoacidosis happens when there is an unusually abnormal state of ketones in the blood expedited by an unregulated biochemical response. This by and large happens in individuals determined to have Type 1 diabetes who can't deliver insulin all alone. Wholesome ketosis is a managed procedure that enables enough insulin to stay in the blood to balance the level of ketones which will keep an ostensibly solid individual from creating Ketoacidosis.

The main courses for somebody following the Ketogenic diet to create Ketoacidosis are:

1. In the event that they are in starvation mode for a while, this won't happen with an appropriately figured feast design.

2. On the off chance that they perform delayed times of greatly high force work out.

3. On the off chance that they are incessant heavy drinkers who enjoy extraordinary gorges

As should be obvious, wholesome ketosis isn't risky when an appropriately planned and took after Ketogenic supper plan is set up. It is a characteristic metabolic process that is superbly ok for any individual who isn't a diabetic who needs insulin or an extreme alcoholic.

What Should I Know & Do Before Starting?

Similarly as with any diet, there are a couple of things that you should know and do before beginning.

As a matter of first importance, be quiet with yourself. You may encounter symptoms as you change your metabolism. You may likewise encounter starting fast weight reduction took after by a level. Simply don't be demoralized, it's simply your body acclimating to the new sum and sort of energy being given.

Second, converse with your doctor to be sure that starting a specific way of life, for example, the Ketogenic diet is for you. You would prefer not to imperil your wellbeing during the time spent endeavoring to enhance it.

Furthermore, third, comprehend what you may involvement and how to facilitate any side effects you may need to manage.

Check with Your Physician

Most therapeutic specialists are not prepared in sustenance and likely don't comprehend the contrasts between nourishing ketosis and Ketoacidosis. While Ketoacidosis is dangerous it is exceptionally uncommon that it happens in individuals not determined to have Type 1 diabetes, which can't create insulin.

There is a lot of misdirecting data out there that has been instructed since the 1960s. Most restorative experts have a tendency to not offer counsel that is the opposite is for the most part acknowledged. If so with your doctor, don't be shocked in the event that they can't discover a reason (other than your new way of life) for your weight reduction and general wellbeing change.

Who Should Not Start a Ketogenic Diet?

While the Ketogenic diet has been shown to be safe for nearly everyone to follow, there are still certain people who should not follow this lifestyle. The first list is rather technical but it will help your physician determine if this lifestyle is healthy and safe for you.

People with Metabolic Conditions

- Type 1 Diabetes

- Primary Carnitine Deficiency

- Carnitine palmitoyltransferase (CPT) Type 1 or 2 deficiencies

- Carnitine translocase deficiency

- Beta-oxidation defects

- Mitochondrial 3-hydroxy 3-methylglutaryl CoA synthase (mHMGS) deficiency

- Long-, Medium-, & short-chain acyl dehydrogenase deficiency (LCAD), (MCAD), & (SCAD)

- Long- & Medium-chain 3 hydroxyacyl-CoA deficiency

- Pyruvate caboxylase deficiency

- Porphyria

People with certain Medical Conditions

- Pancreatitis

- Gall Bladder disease

- Impaired liver function

- Malnutrition

- Gastric bypass surgery

- Abdominal tumors

- Impaired gastric motility (this can be due to cancer treatment and medications)

- Kidney failure

- If you are pregnant or breastfeeding

Advantages and disadvantages of the Ketogenic Diet

Changing your dietary patterns to the Ketogenic diet isn't simple at first. In any case, once you are adjusted to this new way of life you will end up feeling vastly improved and more advantageous therefore.

Keep in mind that these reactions are just transitory and will last from a couple of days up to about a month. On the off chance that you comprehend your physical responses you will have the capacity to figure out how to limit them which will keep you from a portion of the wretchedness caused via starch withdrawal.

How about we get the bad news over with before we go ahead to the advantages of following the Ketogenic diet

Side Effects

Frequent urination

> ➤ As you begin to burn up the stored glycogen in your body, your kidneys will begin getting rid of excess water. For every gram of glycogen stored in your muscles, 3-4 grams of water is also stored. That's a lot of water to get rid of.

Fatigue, Dizziness, Muscle Cramps & Headache

> ➤ As you discharge abundance water it is a given that you will lose electrolytes too; Like, sodium, potassium and magnesium.

> ➤ Weakness and unsteadiness are more typical of the reactions yet can be maintained a strategic distance from by getting enough substitution electrolytes.

> ➤ Utilizing ocean salt to season your nourishment alongside a light salt that is potassium based will help you to supplant those minerals you are losing.

> ➤ 400mg Magnesium citrate supplements each prior night bed will shield you from creating muscle issues.

Hypoglycemia "Also known as low blood sugar"

> ➤ In the event that you've been eating a high carbohydrate diet your body is utilized to a specific measure of insulin coasting around in your circulatory system. When you diminish your starch consumption you may encounter a couple of scenes of low glucose before your body adjusts to the new way of life.

Constipation

- ➢ Constipation is one more of the more typical symptoms of the Ketogenic diet. It is generally because of drying out and salt misfortune however it can likewise be because of eating excessively numerous nuts or a magnesium irregularity.

- ➢ This can be lightened by adjusting your calcium admission, drinking more water and decreasing the measure of nuts you expend.

Sugar Cravings

- ➢ There is a two days up to a three week transition period where you may find yourself experiencing intense sugar cravings. How long this side effect will last is dependent upon how long and how much is your intake from carbohydrate.

- ➢ You can ease these cravings by doing one of the following things:

    1. Eat around four ounces of protein

    2. Take a walk.

    3. Take a B complex vitamin supplements.

    4. Distract yourself

- ➢ Sugar cravings last about an hour so if you can take your mind off it, you will be able to outlast the craving.

Diarrhea

- ➢ This side effect is very common and will resolve itself after a few days.

- ➢ Take an anti-diarrheal or use a teaspoon of sugar-free Metamucil just before your meals until the loose stools stop occurring.

Sleep Changes

- ➢ This reaction varies from individual to individual.

- ➢ It might be an indication that you are encountering lessened insulin or serotonin levels. It can likewise be an indication of histamine prejudice.

- If you get yourself not ready to stay unconscious, you can have a go at eating a nibble just before bed containing protein with a little starch in it.

- You can likewise take a stab at taking a melatonin supplement to enable you to fall and stay unconscious.

Kidney Stones

- Kidney stones are extremely uncommon in individuals following a Ketogenic diet. Be that as it may, it is important to say it just in the event that you are one of the uncommon people who encounter this reaction.

- Be certain to address your specialist before taking any potassium citrate supplement on the off chance that you have kidney or circulatory strain issues.

Low T3 Thyroid Hormone levels

- This isn't really a terrible symptom. It's progressively a specific of a characteristic result of getting into ketosis. It occurs with the more traditional diets also.

- Your body will turn out to be more delicate to the T3 hormone levels so you don't require to such an extent.

Heart palpitations

- There are a few reasons why you may encounter this reaction.

- You may have a regularly low pulse.

- You may require a multivitamin with selenium and zinc and additionally a magnesium supplement.

- It might be because of transient hypoglycemia.

- You may have an electrolyte unevenness or be got dried out.

- You might expend excessively MCT oil, for example, coconut oil. You ought to incorporate margarine, olive oil and creature fats too.

➢ You may require higher protein consumption. Take a stab at including an extra 5-10 grams to your diet.

Hair loss

➢ This side effect isn't related just to the Ketogenic diet. It is possible with any major change in your diet. And it is not happening for all of people who go for diet

➢ Once your insulin levels normalize the hair loss will stop and you should begin to find your hair to be thicker and fuller as it becomes healthier.

Benefits of Going Keto

Lack of hunger

- Ketones diminish your craving.

- Beneficial fats are extremely fulfilling.

- You may wind up neglecting to eat which might stun on the off chance that you battle with nourishment fixation.

Lower blood pressure

- Be certain to counsel with your specialist in the event that you are taking any blood pressure prescriptions since you may feel bleary eyed from an excessive amount of pharmaceutical while on the Ketogenic diet.

Lower cholesterol levels

- Cholesterol is produced using overabundance glucose so when you eat fewer carbohydrates your cholesterol levels will drop.

- Increased HDL levels likewise happen in light of the fact that you will eat more soaked fats, which is something worth being thankful for.

- Decreased triglycerides will happen in light of the fact that they are firmly attached to the measure of carbohydrates you expend.

Lower blood sugar and insulin levels

- With less sugar intake, less insulin will glide in your circulatory system.

- HbA1c will likewise diminish which shows you are apt to a lesser extent a hazard for coronary illness.

Increased energy

- Even in the event that you encounter exhaustion as a side effect, once you adjust to the Ketogenic diet you will locate the interminable weariness side effects subsiding.

Less joint pain and stiffness

> This is one of the well known side effects you will experience by following the Ketogenic diet.

> It is known that grain-based food increases inflammation and causes many chronic illnesses that overweight people suffer from.

Reduce the blurriness

> Since the brain is no less than half fat by weight; it bodes well that the fatter you eat the better your mind can look after itself.

Stabilized sleep patterns

> Sleep apnea has been connected to grain utilization and in addition the acid reflux that can be caused by a high starch diet.

> You will never again feel the requirement for those late evening snoozes that can botch up your circadian beat.

Weight loss

> This is the most widely recognized reactions of following a Ketogenic diet.

> As your metabolism repairs itself you will end up dropping pounds and crawls as you get more beneficial all the while.

> After the underlying quick weight reduction you may wind up at a level. This way of life will enable you to alter your suppers to keep getting in shape.

> Coupled with a sensible exercise routine you will have the capacity to lose more weight while constructing and conditioning muscle and still not feel hungry.

Relief from gastric symptoms

> High carbohydrates diets are regularly the guilty parties in the event that you experience the ill effects of acid reflux, heartburn and GERD.

- ➢ Symptoms will diminish or vanish out and out when following the Ketogenic diet. In the event that despite everything you encounter indigestion and reflux, dispense with tomatoes and talk with your doctor to establish that your irritate bladder is working appropriately.

- ➢ You will discover a lessening in gas and bloating as the lower utilization of grains and sugars kills the aging that happens in your small digestive organs.

Oral health improvements

- ➢ Sugar is known to change the acidity level (pH) of your mouth and causes tooth decay. After a few months following the Ketogenic diet you will find that any gingivitis you might be experiencing will decrease or disappear. Check with your dentist for any damage that may remain.

Increased serotonin and dopamine levels

- ➢ Ketone bodies are known to settle your body's neurotransmitters. This will bring about less emotional episodes enabling you to feel better about yourself and your life by and large.

- ➢ It is obscure right now whether individuals taking particular serotonin reuptake inhibitors (SSRIs) should keep taking those drugs or in the event that they will have the capacity to expel that prescription from their every day schedule.

As the rundowns above show, the obnoxious reactions are brief and the advantages you will understand by changing to the Ketogenic way of life are certainly justified regardless of the exertion.

Counting Macros vs. Calories?

In case you're grabbing this book to take in more about the Ketogenic diet at that point you've most likely catch wind of something many refer to as 'macros' or macronutrients. That is what we will talk about in this segment alongside regardless of whether you ought to check macros or calories. On the off chance that you get the extents of macros right, it will make the diet less demanding to take after where simply confining calories may make you come up short.

Lamentably, traditional diets for the most part don't consider what you are eating, just the calories you are devouring. Bit control can work for some time, however unless you are eating the correct sustenance that will abandon you fulfilled, inevitably your poise will separate. This is the thing that prompts gorging and abandoning a diet inside and out.

In the event that you focus on tallying your macronutrients as opposed to the measure of calories you are taking in, you will wind up eating a greater amount of the correct nourishments. This will help you to adhere to your diet all the more effectively and you may find that you can permit yourself a couple of additional grams of carbohydrates if that happens to be one of your totally most loved nourishments.

What Are Macros?

Macros, or macronutrients, are what we expend that gives energy to our cells. There are three important for people; carbohydrates, fats and proteins. Each of these macronutrients gives us energy when they are separated. This energy comes as calories.

Every gram of carbohydrates and proteins will be separated amid assimilation and give 4 calories. Fats, in any case, give 9 calories to every gram separated by our systems.

Proteins

Protein is related with building muscle tissue. Nonetheless it is the principle part in every one of the organs and tissues of your body, hair and chemicals that your body utilizes once a day. It is comprised of amino acids that are important for the best possible working of our bodies however we can make some of them for ourselves. Lamentably, there are nine amino acids that you should get from the nourishments we eat. These are called fundamental amino acids and are discovered only in meats.

Carbohydrates

You can actually do without carbohydrates yet in the event that you cut it out of your diet totally, your body should locate the little measure of glucose your cerebrum needs from protein. Separating protein into glucose really utilizes more energy than it gives so a little sugar in your diet is something to be thankful for. Simply don't try too hard!

Fats

Fats are regularly insulted in light of the fact that they are calorie-thick nourishments. Be that as it may, they are vital for typical real capacities. Fats make up the foundation of the vast majority of the hormones our body produces, encompasses each nerve to help secure tissues and lead driving forces, and makes our skin and hair solid and solid.

There are various sorts of fats that we at present have in our diets; immersed, monounsaturated, polyunsaturated, Trans fat, thus some more. The ones you should be worried about are Omega-3 and Omega-6 unsaturated fats. Both are essential for feeling solid however Omega-6 fats are considerably less demanding to get than the Omega-3. An overdose of Omega-6 unsaturated fats will bring about an expansion in aggravation in your joints and muscles. In case you're cautious of how you adjust those two fats, you will feel greatly improved and remain on the track to a more sound life.

Does Counting Calories on Keto Help?

You may have heard or perused that you don't have to count calories when you are following a Ketogenic diet. Be that as it may, that is not by any stretch of the imagination genuine. You don't need to count calories while following a Ketogenic diet, however doing as such can enable you to get all that you need out of your new way of life.

Consider checking calories while on Keto as another apparatus in your stockpile against your weight and to enable you to get solid once more. There are numerous sites that will enable you to decide the quantity of calories you take in as is normally done. With a specific end goal to use the Ketogenic diet and calorie considering a double instrument to get in shape, essentially lessen the measure of calories taken in by 500 and utilize the rest of the calorie consider your breaking point. Notwithstanding, you ought to recall that you don't have to take in that numerous calories.

For instance,

Mara a 42 year old female weighs 282 pounds is 5' 7" and has a stationary way of life. She would need to take in around 2300 calories to keep up her weight. On the off chance that she diminished that sum by 500 calories for each day to 1800, she would lose around 1 pound for each week once the underlying water weight is no more. In any case, on the Ketogenic diet Mara may never achieve that 1800 calories for each day in the event that she eats the correct mix of sustenance to keep her inclination full and fulfilled. This will convert into higher weight reduction every week the more distant from that 1800 calorie constrain she remains.

The vegetables you eat while on the Ketogenic diet will furnish you with fiber to feel full more, the protein and fat will offer you the satiation that shields you from feeling hungry and you'll encounter a higher metabolic rate which will make you consume more calories. Due to the satiated inclination subsequent to eating, you will normally confine your caloric admission so you can get in shape somewhat quicker than you would on a traditional diet.

Weight Loss & Muscle Building

A great many people who start following a Ketogenic way of life won't be the individuals who are as of now genuinely fit and have a ton of muscles as of now. Be that as it may, that doesn't imply that you won't not get to that point once you have become near your optimal weight and your coveted wellbeing level.

Once your body is completely adjusted to this new diet and you have lost as much weight as important to feel more invigorated you will have the capacity to alter your menus to oblige building quality and muscle too. When you achieve the point in the 'standard' Ketogenic diet where you crave constructing and conditioning muscle is ideal for you, you will have the capacity to change the diet to what is called 'focused on' or 'repeating'. Both of those renditions of the Ketogenic diet permit more sugar utilization so you can take in enough glucose to nourish your muscles without thumping yourself out of ketosis.

The focused on Ketogenic diet enables you to take in additional carbohydrates around your activity times. This diet is a tradeoff between the standard Ketogenic diet which we have been talking about and the patterned Ketogenic diet that will be depicted shortly. This type of the diet enables you to play out a high power exercise without dropping out of ketosis for a drawn out stretch of time. The admission of more carbohydrates previously an exercise is advantageous in light of the fact that you will have the glucose important for your muscles to work yet all that additional glucose is scorched off amid your exercise so your metabolism isn't changed for more than the 30 minutes or with the goal that your exercise takes. The TKD is for learner or irregular exercisers since it permits a slight increment in sugar allow yet keep you in ketosis without a stun to your framework.

The recurrent Ketogenic diet is for further developed athletic mentors and weight lifters. This shape is utilized for most extreme muscle building. Nonetheless, you may wind up increasing some muscle to fat ratio. This is on the grounds that it is anything but difficult to indulge on this type of the diet notwithstanding the greatly draining exercises you will do on this diet. The CKD has a tendency to make them take after the standard Ketogenic diet for 5 or 6 days took after by 1 or 2 days of high starch eating. The reason this doesn't work for novices is that it can take up to 3 weeks for your body to go completely into ketosis. The objective of this type of the way of life is to briefly change out of ketosis with a specific end goal to refill the measure of glycogen in the muscles to help the extreme exercise amid your next cycle. Keep in mind, on the off chance that you do this kind of diet, that you should totally drain the measure of glycogen amid your instructional meeting. The force of your preparation will rely upon the measure of carbohydrates to take in amid your carbo-loading stage.

Is it Possible Not to Lose Weight on a Ketogenic Diet?

This isn't only a level where you have been getting more fit however the misfortunes have decreased or halted through and through for a week or something like that. This is on the off chance that where you are really not shedding pounds and thinking that it's hard to get into ketosis OR you've been tailing it and something has happened to make it difficult for you to keep to your new way of life. These things can be pressure, the occasions, or even extend of time where you were welcomed out more than once every week.

The short response to this inquiry is yes, it is conceivable that you will encounter an absence of weight reduction while on a Ketogenic diet. In any case, there are a few purposes for this and the greater part of them can be managed by making a few changes in accordance with your menu design and way of life.

You might eat an excessive number of carbohydrates.

- ➢ Decrease your carb admission.

- ➢ Increase the measure of coconut oil in your diet. Coconut oil is a medium chain triglyceride and is all the more effortlessly absorbable and utilized for prompt energy needs.

You might eat excessively or too little protein.

- ➢ Protein is an extremely fulfilling macronutrient.

- ➢ Eating too little protein will prompt muscle misfortune.

- ➢ Eating an excess of protein will prompt an expansion in glycogen in your cells which will show you out of ketosis.

Undermining carbs

> You should be exceptionally restrained and tally each and every carb that you eat.

> Anti-building up specialists are utilized as a part of numerous flavors, table salt and other heating things like preparing powder, preparing pop and cocoa. Other sustenance added substances like emulsifiers/stabilizers, thickeners and gelling operators are likewise regularly sugar based.

> If you end up snacking all over, you should decide whether you are really eager or on the off chance that it is out of propensity.

You might eat an excessive number of fats.

> Yes, it's a high fat diet. In any case, that doesn't mean you can eat 5000 calories worth of fats and hope to get more fit.

> Calories aren't as large an arrangement in the Ketogenic diet inasmuch as you are getting the right measures of all the macronutrients, however do know about the amount you are taking in.

> You might devour the wrong sorts of fats too. Make certain to take in just useful fats while on the Ketogenic diet.

You might take in an excessive number of counterfeit sweeteners (artificial sweeteners).

> Be mindful that any Ketogenic formula may call for Stevia or Erythritol for sweetening. These can cause longings which can influence you to quit getting thinner.

> Artificial sweeteners frequently contain against building up operators which add to your sugar admission. These are not entirely obvious.

> Chewing gum, mints, hack syrups and other sustenance things or meds can contain counterfeit sweeteners and ought to be maintained a strategic distance from at whatever point conceivable.

Extreme dairy and nuts

> Milk is from time to time incorporated into a Ketogenic diet design since it contains high measures of lactose which will be changed straightforwardly into glucose amid processing.

> Limit your cheddar and yogurt admission to lessen the measure of dairy you are expending.

> Nuts are regularly incorporated into a Ketogenic diet however dependably in restricted sums because of the high caloric substance.

> Too much dairy and nuts can show you out of ketosis since they are calorie-thick nourishments and are anything but difficult to enjoy.

You might be near your objective weight.

> Losing weight turns out to be more troublesome the nearer you get to your optimal weight.

> To keep getting in shape once you have achieved this level, you may need to alter your macronutrient admission or increment your activity power, or both.

You might be under more worry than you might suspect.

> When you are focused on your body will create more cortisol which is the thing that influences your body to store fat and make shedding pounds more troublesome.

> Stress is connected to hypothyroidism and additionally adrenal issues that can influence your metabolism.

- ➤ Gentle exercise and daylight will facilitate the measure of pressure you are under. On the off chance that you feel yourself getting to be plainly pushed, go for a stroll outside for around 20 minutes and you will end up resting easy and the want to pressure eat will vanish.

Your circadian rhythms might be upset.

- ➤ Sleep is basic for long haul weight reduction.

- ➤ Try to rest before midnight and get in the vicinity of 7 and 9 hours of rest every night.

- ➤ Unless you get yourself greedy when you wake early in the day, attempt to abstain from eating in the 3 hours before you rest. In the event that you should have a sleep time nibble, ensure it has adjusted of fats, protein and carbs with the goal that you won't drop out of ketosis.

You may practice excessively.

- ➤ Too much exercise can be as terrible for you as insufficient when you are in the getting thinner stage.

- ➤ Remember that muscle measures more than fat so regardless of whether you are following your diet entirely and still not getting more fit, this might be the reason. This should just happen on the off chance that you are past the getting in shape stage and moving into the muscle conditioning and building stage.

- ➤ Adjust your full scale admission to suit your activity schedule.

You may have a thyroid or adrenal issue that you have never been determined to have or been tried for.

- ➤ Consult with your doctor for testing to be sure you are not managing a thyroid or adrenal brokenness.

- Low-sugar diets are not proposed for anybody with hypothyroidism or adrenal ailment.

You might encounter an absence of leptin creation.

- Leptin is a hormone put off by fat cells that advises the body to quit eating.

- Elevated leptin levels demonstrate satiety subsequent to eating.

- As you shed pounds you will have less fat cell so your body might not have sufficiently high leptin levels to flag satiety.

- This can be cured by eating sustenance rich in both fat and protein.

You might utilize manufactured sweeteners that contain sugar alcohols.

- Sweeteners, for example, Stevia, Swerve, Erythritol and chicory root don't contain sugar alcohols so are better for use in a Ketogenic formula.

- Products marked as 'low-fat' are regularly brimming with included sugars. The purpose for this is something must be added to influence it to taste great since fat is the thing that conveys season. In the event that fat is removed from a sustenance item, something different must be utilized to convey the flavor and the optional bearer is a starch.

You may not get enough water and electrolytes.

- Water is crucial for fat misfortune so you have to ensure you are legitimately hydrated.

- Water stifles the craving and causes you use fat.

- Proper admission of electrolytes, for example, magnesium, potassium and sodium help to shield you from holding water and additionally ensuring that your muscles work appropriately.

➤ The perfect measure of electrolytes will likewise shield your muscles from cramping. The poisons developed by issues can cause longings for both salt and carbohydrates due to the aggravation encompassing the confined muscles.

What Can I Do If I faced steady state?

Reaching a steady state is not altogether unexpected on the Ketogenic diet. It happens in any kind of diet that you might choose to follow.

When you start to lose weight and get in shape, your metabolism will decay. This makes you consume fewer calories than you did at your heavier weight. The slower your metabolism, the slower you will get thinner regardless of whether you eat a similar number of calories that had initially helped you get in shape. At the point when the calories you consume approach the quantity of calories you eat, you will achieve a level.

There are a couple of ways that you can get through a steady with the goal that you can keep getting in shape until the point when you are prepared to start a delicate exercise and muscle conditioning schedule.

Eat more fiber

- You can add psyllium husk to about any sustenance. It is utilized as a thickener and also to influence Ketogenic to bread.

- Additional fiber will enable you to feel full more and will diminish the measure of nourishment you are eating.

- Make sense of your state of mind toward sustenance. Recognizing what rouses you to eat will help you to make your arrangement to conquer those useless inclinations.

- If you are on edge, anxious or discouraged, you may find that you eat to rest easy. This is called passionate craving.

- Emotional hunger goes ahead all of a sudden. It is regularly overpowering and feels earnest, perhaps agonizing.

- Emotional hunger influences you to pine for particular nourishments, particularly comfort sustenance. Sadly, those yearnings are frequently for sugary or greasy nourishments. Greasy nourishments on the Ketogenic diet are not generally terrible for you but rather when it is candidly determined the greasy sustenance you may desire aren't really the helpful fats supported on your Keto diet.

- Emotional hunger isn't fulfilled when your stomach is full. You will regularly get yourself awkwardly full which will prompt acid reflux, indigestion, acrid stomach, looseness of the bowels or stoppage and now and again regurgitating.

- Emotional hunger doesn't originate from your stomach since you are longing for something in light of the surface, the taste or the possess an aroma similar to the sustenance.

- If you are inclined to passionate yearning, you will regularly feel regretful in light of the fact that you realize that you are not eating for healthful reasons. Lament and disgrace are additionally part of the feelings that happen after passionate eating which can prompt proceeded with enthusiastic eating.

- Emotional hunger is the most hard to overcome yet it is as yet conceivable. Keep in mind that most passionate eating is caused by upsetting sentiments yet it can likewise be utilized as a reward for an achievement or while commending an occasion. You can do any of the accompanying to escape the propensity for eating when your feelings are included.

- Distinguish your trigger. Is it true that you are focused? Is it true that you are stuffing or hushing awkward feelings? It is safe to say that you are exhausted or excessively worn out? Is it a propensity from youth to remunerate yourself for something you've done? Do you get a handle on anxious when you're with companions?

- Occupy yourself when you end up needing to eat inwardly. Call a companion or relative. Walk your canine or play with your feline. Consume anxious energy by moving to your main tune or taking a lively walk. Appreciate some tea or glass of wine in a hot shower with calming oils. Read a book, investigate outside, deal with a leisure activity you appreciate.

- Take 30 minutes for yourself consistently. Exercise. Ponder. On the off chance that you are religious, perused your heavenly book and ask. Sleep. Invest energy with individuals who improve your life.

- If you are rash you may need to expel allurements from your home and take somebody with you when you go shopping for food to let you know 'no' when you get to the checkout counter.

- If you don't focus on what you eat then you will need to evade circumstances where nourishment is accessible while you are accomplishing something unique, for example, staring at the TV.

- Engage in fasting and high force practice every so often.

Intermittent Exercise & Fasting

- High power and discontinuous exercise and fasting can break a level and get you back on the weight reduction track. Fasting now and again regards help to rinse your assortment of developed poisons and to kick off your metabolism when it comes to the heart of the matter of leveling. Discontinuous high force exercise can likewise kick off your metabolism by enhancing your glucose resilience and copying abundance calories. Due to the force any glycol that remaining parts developed in the muscles will be drained which will help you to stay in ketosis. Since glycol expects water to be put away then you will have more water-weight that will be lost too.

Intermittent High Intensity Exercise

- This is an activity method where you exchange extreme anaerobic exercise with short recuperation periods.

- One impact is that you will consume more calories in less time contrasted with low power exercises which are for the most part high-impact works out.

- 15-20 minute exercises with a 5 minute warm up and a 5 minute chill off to abstain from cramping.

- The thought behind anaerobic exercise is to make your muscles feel exhausted in a brief timeframe. The following are some proposed practices that will achieve this inside that 10 minute time of extraordinary exercise.

Heavy weight lifting

- You should just have the capacity to lift this weight 3 to 6 times before your muscles feel exhausted.

High speed burpees

- These ought to be executed as fast as conceivable so they are anaerobic instead of oxygen consuming. To play out a burpee take after the headings underneath.

- Remain with your hands at your sides.

- Crouch and place your hands on the floor about shoulder width separated.

- Bounce your feet back with the goal that you are in the push up position.

- Play out a push up.

- Hop your feet back to your hands so you are hunched down once more.

- Jump into the air.

- Land with your knees twisted and rehash

- Perceive what number of you can perform in 60 seconds and rest for 60 seconds between redundancies. Proceed until the point that your muscles feel exhausted or 10 minutes.

- In the event that the push up or the jumps are excessively strenuous, you can discard those until the point when you are better ready to achieve them.

Sprinting

- This requires a full scale exertion which makes it anaerobic.

- On the off chance that you don't approach a track or other level zone to run, you can do runs set up.

- Start by running set up to get your beat.

- Lift your knees with the goal that your thighs are parallel to the floor. Pump your arms vivaciously.

- Pick up the pace until the point when you are going as quick as possible.

- Continue for 30 to 60 seconds.

- Rest for 60 seconds and rehash for residual time

Double-under Jump Rope

- This is a high-force hop rope practice that is a compelling exercise regularly utilized by boxers.

- Begin by bouncing rope typically to get used to the development.

- When you feel prepared, bounce somewhat higher and increment the speed you are turning the rope.

- Keep hopping rope ordinarily until the point when you are prepared to do another twofold under.

- When you have idealized your strategy at this activity, you can start to do numerous twofold unders consecutive.

- On the off chance that you are simply starting twofold unders, bounce rope with irregular twofold unders for 3 minutes, Rest for 30 seconds before playing out a moment 3 minute set

- On the off chance that you are skilled at twofold unders, perform 10 out of a column, rest 30 seconds, perform 20 of every a line, rest 30 seconds, and after that perform 30 out of a line with 30 second rest periods until the point that your activity time constrain is up.

Kettle bell swings

- You can play out this activity utilizing a solitary dumbbell or an overwhelming weight in a pack that won't tear.

- This activity targets hamstrings; bring down back, upper back and glutes.

- Keeping in mind the end goal to play out this activity, take after the bearings underneath.

- Hold the weight in the two submits front of your hips.

- Bend your knees marginally and push your butt in reverse to bring down the weight to hang between your knees.

- Shove your hips forward and utilize that energy to swing the weight upward to bear tallness. Keep your arms straight however control the weight to shield it from swinging too far.

- Let the weight swing back to knee stature and rehash.

- Try to complete 15 swings for each minute.

- Do not permit your back to round as this can cause bring down back damage.

Intermittent Fasting

- This is precisely as it sounds. You will quick in the vicinity of 14 and 36 hours with an exceptionally strict 'sustaining window'. For the more drawn out quick periods, you can part your 'window' in two if fundamental.

    a. If you quick for 14 hours, your 'nourishing window' is 2-3 hours.

    b. If you quick for 24 hours, your 'nourishing window' is 4-6 hours.

    c. If you quick for 36 hours, your 'nourishing window' is 6-8 hours.

- The thought is that you will eat as much as you need amid your 'sustaining window' yet when you are in your 'fasting period' you won't take in anything with caloric esteem.

Feeding Window

- Attempt to come to your macronutrient focus without limiting yourself yet ensure you just eat to satiety.

  a. It may not be conceivable to come to your macronutrient target and that is superbly worthy.

  b. Eat the majority of your protein. Keep in mind that on the off chance that you eat less protein than required, you may lose muscles, diminish your metabolic rate and wind up consuming less muscle versus fat.

  c. Eat as a lot of your fats as important to wind up noticeably fulfilled

- Carbohydrates are the slightest vital to expend amid this nourishing window. In the event that you incorporate carbohydrates, at that point keep your admission to be less than 20 grams.

Fasting Window

- When fasting, you will just expend fluids with zero caloric as well as nourishing worth.

- Water is clearly permitted.

- Dark espresso or tea sweetened with Stevia or erythritol are permitted.

- While neither High Intensity Intermittent Exercise nor Intermittent Fasting are ideal for weight reduction, they are both great devices to use to get through a determined level. When you have returned to shedding pounds you can alter your macronutrient and caloric admission

Approved Foods, Meal Plans and Other Important Information

This segment will give you a considerable measure of essential data that may appear somewhat overpowering. Try not to give it a chance to demoralize you when you see numerous sustenance on the 'totally keep away from' list, particularly in the event that they are some of your top choices. You truly can make this work for you.

What Foods Can You Eat?

Fats

Avocado Oil

Almond Oil

Beef Tallow; should be from grass fed cattle

Butter; organic if possible

Chicken Fat

Duck Fat

Ghee; goat butter with the milk solids removed

Lard; NOT hydrogenated, organic if possible

Macadamia Oil

Mayonnaise; read the label to be sure it has no carbs in it

Olive Oil

Sesame Oil

Flaxseed Oil

Hemp Oil

Coconut Oil

Coconut Butter

Coconut Cream; concentrated, organic

Proteins

Beef

Lamb

Veal

Goat

Wild game

Pork; read the label of ham, sausage and bacon to avoid added sugar

Chicken

Turkey

Duck

Goose

Game birds

Anchovies

Calamari

Catfish

Cod

Flounder

Halibut

Herring

Mackerel

Mahi-mahi

Salmon; canned is allowed, read the label for added sugar or carb-fillers

Sardines

Scrod

Sole

Snapper

Trout

Tuna; canned is allowed, read the label for added sugar or carb-fillers

Clams

Crab

Lobster

Scallops

Shrimp

Squid

Mussels

Oysters

Whole eggs; cooked in a variety of ways

Peanut Butter; read the label for carbohydrates, natural is best

Tempeh; read the label for carbohydrates

Tofu; read the label for carbohydrates

Edamame; read the label for carbohydrates

Whey protein powders; be very careful about the contents of the product, determine the amount of added sugars and fillers that may be included

Vegetables

Alfalfa sprouts

Asparagus

Avocado; Hass is best for eating

Bamboo shoots

Bean sprouts

Beet greens

Bell peppers *

Bok choy

Broccoli

Brussels sprouts

Cabbage

Carrots *

Cauliflower

Celery

Celery root

Chard

Chives

Collard greens

Cucumbers

Dandelion greens

Pickles; dill

Garlic

Kale

Leeks

Arugula

Boston butter lettuce

Chicory

Endive

Escarole

Fennel

Radicchio

Romaine

Mushrooms

Olives

Onions *

Radishes

Sauerkraut; be careful of added sugar unless making it yourself

Scallions

Shallots

Snow peas

Spinach

Summer squash *

Tomatoes *

Turnips

Zucchini

Water chestnuts

* These vegetables are higher in carbohydrates so intake should be limited.

Dairy Products

Heavy whipping cream

Sour cream; full fat, read labels for additives and fillers

Cottage cheese; full fat

Cheddar

Swiss

Colby

Monterey Jack

Provolone

Munster

Gouda

Farmer cheese

Blue cheese

Cream cheese

Mascarpone

Yogurt; unsweetened, full fat, Greek, limit how much you eat due to the higher carb content

Nuts & Seeds

It is best to soak and/or roast nuts and seeds to get rid of any possible anti-nutrients they may contain. Since they are very high in carbs you will need to limit your intake. Too many nuts and seeds can cause increased inflammation so you should not depend upon them for all of your protein needs. Nuts and seeds can also cause a disruption in you moods.

Macadamias

Pecans

Almonds

Walnuts

Cashews

Pistachios

Chestnuts

Almond flour

Peanuts

Pumpkin seeds

Sunflower seeds

Sesame seeds

Hemp seeds

Chia seeds

Beverages

All beverages should be unsweetened. Use artificial sweeteners sparingly. Be certain that all beverages are decaffeinated since caffeine can increase blood sugar.

Bone broth

Decaffeinated coffee

Decaffeinated tea

Herbal tea

Water

Flavored seltzer water

Lemon juice

Lime juice

Almond milk

Hazelnut milk

Cashew milk

Coconut milk

Soy milk

Hemp milk

Fruits, Spices & Miscellaneous

Most fruits should be avoided since they are high in carbohydrates in the form of fructose. However, there are some berries that can be enjoyed in small amounts once in a while.

Blueberries

Strawberries

Raspberries

Cranberries

Blackberries

Any flavor that you don't crush yourself will contain carbohydrates. Monetarily made flavor blends as a rule contain included sugar. For salting dishes, you should utilize ocean salt as opposed to general iodized salt which is frequently joined with powdered dextrose to forestall amassing. Notwithstanding, there are a few flavors that have irrelevant measures of carbs included that you will discover in numerous Ketogenic formulas. In spite of those carbs being irrelevant doesn't mean you shouldn't tally them. There are sites that enable you to put in your total formula, including flavors, and the site will figure the greater part of your macros and in addition calories which will enable you to incorporate those 'unimportant' carbs.

Black pepper

Basil

Cayenne pepper

Chili powder

Cilantro

Cinnamon

Cumin

Ginger

Cardamom

Bay leaves

Oregano

Parsley

Rosemary

Sage

Thyme

Turmeric

Different things you can appreciate in constrained sums are Japanese Shirataki noodles, pork skins and 85-90% chocolate. Pork skins are a decent substitute for bread scraps yet they are high in protein so you should constrain your utilization of them.

Some Ketogenic formulas, particularly treats, require some type of sweetening and you should be watchful about how much counterfeit sweetener you use since you are attempting to get a more common diet going. That being stated, the best sweeteners to utilize are characteristic like nectar or agave. You simply should be exceptionally watchful about the amount you utilize and take after the formula precisely with the goal that you are not adding excessively numerous carbohydrates to your every day designation.

Foods You Should Absolutely Avoid

Sugars & Sweeteners

Maple syrup

Malt syrup

Treacle

Carob syrup

Brown sugar

Turbinado sugar

White sugar

Confectioners or powdered sugar

Beet sugar

Cane juice

Cane syrup

Caramel

Panela

Panocha

Coconut sugar

Date sugar

Corn syrup

Sorghum

Molasses

Rice syrup

Maltose

Barley malt

Malt-dextrin

Fruit syrups

Fruit juice concentrate

Tapioca syrup

And any food or food additive that ends in -ose.

Grains & Grain Products

Wheat

Barley

Oats

Rye

Sorghum

Tricale

Spelt

Rice

Bread

Muffins

Rolls

Bread crumbs

Waffles

Pancakes

Pasta

Any commercial cereals; hot and cold

Tortillas

Crackers

Cookies

Tarts

Cakes

Pies

Pretzels

Oatmeal

Cous Cous

Cream of wheat

Quinoa

Kashi

Cornbread

Tamale wrappers

Corn chips

Grits

Polenta

Popcorn

Cornmeal

Fruits, Vegetables & Legumes

Apples

Bananas

Plantains

Pears

Oranges

Grapefruits

Peaches

Apricots

Currents

Cantaloupe

Honeydew Melon

Watermelon

Cherries

Dates

Figs

Gooseberries

Grapes

Raisins

Guava

Mango

Nectarines

Kiwi

Papaya

Plums

Pineapple

Pumpkin

Pomegranates

Potatoes

Sweet potatoes

Hash browns

Potato chips

Tater tots

French fries

Mashed potatoes

Corn

Lima beans

Peas

Okra

Artichokes

Kidney beans

Black beans

Black-eyed peas

Chickpeas

Great northern beans

Vegetable juice concentrate

Lentils

Other Foods You Should Avoid

Canned soups

Canned stews

Processed, boxed 'convenience' foods

Foods listed as 'low-fat', 'low-carb', 'sugar-free', etc. This includes prepared foods and snack bars produced for known HFLC diets like Atkins and South Beach. The reason is that the preservatives tend to be carbohydrate based which can mitigate the benefits of going low-carb.

Beer

Hard liquor

Sweet or dessert wines; dry wines are allowed in limited amounts

Carbonated beverages (aka Soda-pop); both diet and non-diet

Milk; liquid milk contains lactose. Cheese and yogurt is allowed since the fermentation process reduces the amount of lactose in the milk solids.

How Can You Make This Work For You?

Numerous individuals need to take after a Ketogenic diet. You may realize that it is the way of life for you yet you don't know whether you can influence it to work with your bustling timetable. You don't need to be a stay-at-home parent or invest all your energy in the kitchen just to make the suppers either.

With the Ketogenic diet you will choose what sort of nourishments you'll eat and with the web having several destinations that have formulas for this way of life, it ought to be no issue at all to discover dinners you can settle and appreciate in a brief timeframe.

It doesn't make a difference on the off chance that you are the CEO of a Fortune 500 organization or a Kindergarten instructor. In the event that you have to roll out this improvement, you will figure out how to influence it to function. The way of life may not be for everybody, but rather it ought to be.

Determining Your Numbers and Cooking For One

The way to comprehension the Ketogenic way of life and influencing it to work for you by cooking your own sustenance is to recall that you are changing out the carbohydrates in your diet for a higher fat and more direct protein admission.

Fats have extremely constrained impact on glucose levels and insulin creation in your body. Be that as it may, protein affects both of those on the off chance that you eat more than your body requires. The suggested measure of protein that ought to be expended is 0.36 grams for each pound. Lamentably, the normal diet today proposes substantially higher sums than you really require so all that additional protein that isn't separated to the 9 basic amino acids will move toward becoming glucose which is put away as fat. This larger amount of glucose will help the insulin levels in your blood which will slow down the body's capacity to discharge and copy ketones.

The Ketogenic diet design works best when you track the measure of carbs you eat. All Ketogenic designs permit a genuinely expansive scope of grams every day of carbohydrates, in the vicinity of 20 and 60 grams for each day. Nonetheless, it is proposed that in the event that you are simply starting the new way of life you should restrict your sugar admission to close to 20 grams for every day.

The measure of protein you will expend won't be founded on your present weight yet on the weight you need to reach. Because a man weighs 350 pounds, that doesn't mean they will eat at least 120 grams of protein. Your protein admission will be founded on your optimal weight and in addition your sexual orientation and the amount you work out. Keep in mind than men require somewhat more protein than ladies. The individuals who have a modestly dynamic exercise routine likewise require more protein than the individuals who lead a more inactive life.

So how would you decide your rates and the grams of each macronutrient you have to devour on the Ketogenic diet? We should work with two or three cases so you can decide the numbers for yourself.

Example number 1

Dora is a 40 year old woman, 5' 7", 285 pounds and is a secretary who does not exercise on a weekly basis. Her ideal weight is roughly between 120-160 pounds. She chooses to reach the highest end of her ideal weight when starting the Ketogenic diet; 160 pounds.

Protein: 160 X 0.36 = 57.6 grams per day

Dora's intake of protein each day will be rounded up to 58 grams which will be set at 20% protein consumption. This will give her the proper amount of essential amino acids her body needs to function properly without increasing her blood glucose and insulin levels. Once she has her required grams of protein, she will be able to determine her carbohydrate percentage. Let's say that Mary chooses 5% as her carb intake.

Carbohydrate: 58 / 4 = 14.5 grams per day

Dora will round up again to give her 15 grams of carbohydrates per day. Eliminating all grains, most fruits and starchy vegetables will allow her to eat plenty of vegetables and still maintain this minimal intake of carbohydrates.

Now Dora needs to figure out the amount of fats she will consume. It's a bit easier since the remaining 75% of her diet will consist of nutritious and healthy fats, but she still needs to know the grams so that she doesn't overdo and make the Ketogenic diet not work properly for her.

Fats: (58 X 3) + (15 X 3) = 219 grams per day

So this is Dora's Ketogenic 75:20:5 intake; 219 grams of fats, 58 grams of protein and 15 grams of carbohydrates. This is one way for Dora to determine how much she needs to eat each day.

Example Number 2

Dora's doctor is willing to allow her to try this diet and will keep a close watch on her health. However, he has suggested that she combine calorie counting along with the Ketogenic plan. Dora and her doctor have decided that a 1500 calorie diet would allow her to lose weight and still not be hungry while living the Ketogenic lifestyle.

Fats: 1500 X 0.75 = 1125 calories from fat

1125 cal / 9 cal per gram = 125 grams per day

This may seem like a lot of fat to eat per day but you won't be resorting to eating sticks of butter. 1 tablespoon of butter has 11 grams of fat so if you add olive oil, avocados and coconut oil as they appear in your recipes then it won't seem as if you are eating quite that much on a daily basis.

Protein: 1500 X 0.20 = 300 calories from protein

300 / 4 = 75 grams per day

Yes, this amount is more than what was found using the recommended amount per pound of ideal body weight but this will still keep her from losing muscle mass and give her all the amino acids she needs.

Carbohydrate: 1500 X 0.05 = 75 calories from carbs

75 / 4 = 18.75 grams per day

This amount too is slightly more than when using a pure percentage calculation, but Dora has the option of reducing this amount as well if she chooses.

Both of the previous examples will allow Dora to lose weight and begin feeling better. As she slims down and her health returns, the energy this lifestyle offers her will give her the chance to increase her exercise routine.

Whenever you find yourself on steady state while following this lifestyle exactly it is usually an indication that you need to alter your percentages. You may need to increase your protein and exercise routine, which won't be a problem once you start feeling more healthy. If you are increasing your protein you will need to decrease your carbohydrate intake as well. The amount of healthy fats you take in on a daily basis should remain the same with only slight fluctuations as you alter your routines.

If you are also counting calories while following this lifestyle you will need to reduce your caloric intake to continue losing weight If you plateau and have not reached your chosen weight. Simple re-calculate your grams per day with the new calorie amount and adjust your meal plan as needed.

Discovering Meal Plans That Fit Your Life

Finding a supper arrange for that will fit your life is anything but difficult to do in the day and age of the web. Sites swarm with instant dinner designs and countless formulas that can be utilized with the Ketogenic diet.

You have your rates and the suggested grams you ought to expend every day so now there are a couple of things that you have to consider and do as such that you are effective with this way of life.

Get a Carbohydrate counter guide. This is a rundown of what number of carbohydrates in all nourishment that you may experience amid your new way of life. It likewise covers the greater part of the very prepared nourishments that you were eating before going Keto. Monitoring your carbs is the basic piece of this program so a carb counter will enable you to know and see how to do it accurately.

Complete a carb clear. Experience your kitchen and nourishment stockpiling zones. Dispose of all your high carb nourishments, prepared nibble sustenance and any 'complex carbs'. This incorporates anything promoted as 'low carb' since those items can contain concealed carbs that will toss you out of ketosis.

Go shopping. You will need to restock your wash room and icebox with nourishments that will fit your new way of life and enable you to evade allurement. With this new way of life you will end up shopping all the more frequently. Since numerous vegetables keep going for about seven days, you'll need to make sure that you utilize the freshest conceivable create in your formulas.

Consider what you will eat and how to design your suppers. This causes you when you go to the supermarket. On the off chance that you know precisely what you will have for the week, you will be less inclined to just meander and get whatever looks great.

Change your morning schedule. On the off chance that you stop at the coffeehouse while in transit to work and get a bagel with your espresso, make your espresso at home and appreciate it with a few seared eggs.

Drink a lot of water. As you quit taking in carbohydrates your body will begin disposing of overabundance water as your glycogen levels diminish. This can prompt lack of hydration. You may likewise need to drink electrolyte substitution drinks however make sure to tally the carb sums since most games drinks have included sweeteners. Else you can basically add salt to your dinners and take magnesium and potassium supplements.

Consider taking natural supplements. These help support cellular respiration and reduces inflammation by increasing your antioxidant levels.

- Alpha-lipoic acid – 200-600 mg per day

- L-glutamine – 500-1000 mg per day

- CoQ10 – 100-300 mg per day

- Magnesium citrate or malate – 400-600 mg per day

- Potassium – 99 mg per day

- Vitamin C – 500 mg per day

- Vitamin D – 400-2500 IU per day

- Vitamin E – 100 mg per day

- L-Carnitine – 500-1000 mg per day

- A multi-vitamin without iron will give you all the B vitamins you need in addition to what you ingest with each meal.

- Iron is not recommended since bacteria and viruses will use any extra to find a foothold in your intestines to make you ill. Small amounts are necessary and can be found in red meats and some leafy green vegetables but excess amounts can be dangerous.

Purchase Medical Reagent Strips. These are used to check your ketone levels so that you can be sure that you are in nutritional ketosis. You should be able to find either the urine or blood strips in your pharmacy. If you are using the blood ketone strips you will need a special meter which can also be found in your pharmacy.

Monitor your day by day nourishment admission. Keep a diary or spreadsheet that incorporates the measure of nourishment you eat, the macronutrient gram sums and additionally your calories in the event that you are checking those. This will enable you to track how the diet influences you to feel. You can think back and see what works for you.

Try not to thrash yourself for 'deceiving'. Not every person will take after the Ketogenic diet. You will experience your 'old' sustenance at work environment parties, at get together with loved ones or at the occasions. Insofar as you don't scarf down a heated potato or a plate of stew cheddar fries alongside that brew you will be fine. You can limit the likelihood of dropping out of ketosis even at these occasions by eating the parts that you know fit with your diet; serving of mixed greens, meat, cheeses. A couple of additional grams of carbohydrates once won't upset your new way of life all that much. You may need to do 'harm control' the following day to get yourself back on track yet in light of the fact that you are following the Ketogenic way of life, it doesn't mean you need to end up a recluse to do as such.

Toss out your lavatory scale. Truly, dispose of it. Conceal it at any rate. Regardless of whether you began a Ketogenic diet to get in shape, you don't have to center around your weight. Your weight will differ in the vicinity of 1 and 5 pounds each day and measuring yourself consistently without seeing the numbers go down will make you insane! Rather, center on the way you feel and how your garments are fitting. Insofar as your wellbeing is enhancing and your garments are getting looser, you are doing everything right and the new way of life is working.

Insofar as you pick formulas that will take after the rates of fats, proteins and carbohydrates, you will think that its simple to fit Ketogenic into your bustling life schedule. On the off chance that you find that you are running into fundamentally the same as formulas by completing a web seek on Ketogenic formulas; you can simply use formulas from the very much like Paleo diet. In the event that you utilize Paleo formulas you should run the formulas through a carb counter to make sure that you are not taking in too much. The best utilization of

Paleo formulas is to change them into a Keto diet formula which is genuinely simple to do.

In the following part you will discover some example formulas that will demonstrate to you what to search for in a formula. You may likewise get a few thoughts for adjusting suppers that you and your family as of now appreciate with the goal that they are more Ketogenic well disposed.

You Can Enjoy Snacks & Even Dine Out!

While the vast majority on the Ketogenic diet find that they do consummately fine on 2 or 3 dinners every day, others find that they do require bites to keep up that harmony amongst ketosis and not feeling hunger.

This frequently happens when your routine is hindered from your normal calendar. In the event that that is the situation, you can frequently have a couple of things close by to control that craving until the point when you can return home where you can eat your general feast.

You simply should make sure that you are including the macros incorporated your nibble into your day by day allow. The following is a short rundown of things that influence a decent nibble for when you to require some additional lift to your day.

- Cheese – about 2 ounces of mozzarella, cheddar, co-jack in slice or stick form. Be sure to check the label for carbohydrates as well as the fat and protein.

- Sliced ham and cream cheese roll-ups

- Olives

- Nuts

- A boiled egg

- Canned sardines in olive oil or sauce. Again, be certain to check the label for how many grams of carbs, proteins and fats you're adding to your diet and compensate for them.

- Leftover meat from a previous meal

- Boiled or steamed shrimp

- Smoked salmon strips spread with cream cheese

- ½ Haas avocado and half a medium tomato cubed and tossed with mayonnaise

- Beef jerky cured without sugar

- Tuna salad spread on cucumber rounds

In the event that you find that you are continually getting ravenous between dinners you may not eat enough fat and perhaps protein too. You shouldn't fear fat. Increment the measure of gainful fats so you can stay fulfilled and never again require the between dinner snacks.

Some other time that you may feel the Ketogenic diet is awkward is the point at which you are welcomed out to eat with your companions or should go to suppers for business. You shouldn't have any trouble at eateries since you can ask for that the potato, fries or rice be exchanged for a serving of mixed greens or steamed vegetables. You can request additional margarine to spread onto your steak or vegetables which will loan additional flavor and include dampness.

On the off chance that you are basically going out with your companions to a fast food joint or a games bar to watch the amusement, ground sirloin sandwiches or chicken wings are regularly the slightest terrible choice even with the sauces that go ahead the wings. Clearly you ought to maintain a strategic distance from the soda pops and fries. You can simply drink water regardless of whether your companions are enjoying a brew or three, be the assigned driver so everybody returns home securely. Pizza garnishes are alright and the stricter you are with yourself, the less hull you will eat.

This being stated, in the event that you entirely take after your Ketogenic diet each day, it will be to a lesser degree an issue for you to make a couple of special cases when you are welcomed out. If you aren't sure of the expected menu, for example, while heading off to a companion's home for a dinner, you can eat something at home before you clear out. Doing as such will enable you to restrict your segments on the off chance that you find that it is something you ought not have.

Snacks free recipes

Free salty and sweet recipes for you.

Salty snacks

Cucumber mini sandwiches

Enough to make: 4 mini sandwiches

Required time to prepare: 10 minutes

Ingredients:

-   2 cucumbers, sliced into ¼-inch rounds

-   2 tablespoons hummus

-   1 carrot, shredded

-   4 slices turkey ham

-   4 slices cheese

Directions:

Spread the hummus over half of the cucumber slices.

Cut the cheese and ham into squares that fit onto cucumber slices.

Top the hummus with carrots, ham and cheese slice. Repeat until you are out of ingredients.

Top with remaining cucumber slices and serve.

Roasted Brussels sprouts chips

Enough to make: 2 chips

Required time to prepare: 15 minutes

Ingredients:

- 10 Brussels sprouts

- ¼ teaspoon salt

- 1 tablespoon olive oil

Directions:

Preheat oven to 350F.

Carefully split the leaves, making sure not to damage. Toss in a bowl with olive oil and place onto rimmed baking sheet. Season with salt and roast for 10 minutes.

Serve while still warm.

Jalapeno poppers

Enough to make: 4 poppers

Required time to prepare: 15 minutes

Ingredients:

- 16 jalapenos

- 16 slices bacon

- 1 teaspoon salt

- 1 teaspoon paprika

- 4oz. cream cheese

- ¼ cup shredded cheddar cheese

Directions:

Preheat oven to 350F.

Cut bacon in half; cut the jalapenos in half lengthwise.

Mix the cream cheese and cheddar in a bowl.

Fill each jalapeno with cheese mix and wrap around with bacon. Sprinkle with salt and paprika and place into baking dish lined with foil.

Bake the poppers for 25 minutes; serve while still hot.

Pizza fat bomb

Enough to make: 6 bombs

Required time to prepare: 15 minutes

Ingredients:

- 2 tablespoons basil, fresh, chopped

- 4oz. cream cheese

- 14 slices pepperoni, chopped

- 8 black olives, pitted, chopped

- 2 tablespoons sun-dried tomato pesto

- Salt and pepper, to taste

Directions:

In a bowl combine the cream cheese, basil and tomato pesto.

Add the chopped pepperoni and olives. Stir to combine.

Form balls from prepared mixture and serve after on a piece of pepperoni slice.

Chia seed crackers

Enough to make: 36 crackers

Required time to prepare: 45 minutes

Ingredients:

- 3oz. cheddar cheese, shredded

- ½ cup Chia seeds, ground

- ¼ teaspoon paprika

- ¼ teaspoon oregano, dried

- ¼ teaspoon garlic powder

- ¼ teaspoon salt

- ¼ teaspoon black pepper

- 1 ¼ cups water

- 2 tablespoons olive oil

- 2 tablespoons Psyllium Husk

Directions:

In a bowl combine the Chia seeds with Psyllium husk powder, oregano, paprika, garlic powder, salt and black pepper. Mix well.

Add olive oil and mix until you have consistency of wet sand.

Add water and continue mixing until you get solid dough. Stir in grated cheese and knead all with clean hands.

Place the dough onto baking sheet and let it rest for few minute. Cover with second piece of parchment paper and roll out to ¼-inch thickness. Remove top layer of the paper and bake in preheated oven for 35 minutes at 375F. Remove from the oven, cut into desired shape and bake for 5-8 minutes more. Place on the wire rack to cool and serve after.

Cheddar biscuits

Enough to make: 12 biscuits

Required time to prepare: 40 minutes

Ingredients:

- 1 ½ cups almond flour

- 2 eggs

- 4 cups broccoli florets

- ¼ cup coconut oil, melted

- 2 cups cheddar cheese, grated

- 1 teaspoon salt

- 1 teaspoon garlic powder

- 1 teaspoon paprika

- ½ teaspoon baking soda

- ½ teaspoon cider vinegar

Directions:

Preheat oven to 375F and line baking sheet with parchment paper.

Pulse broccoli in food processor until finely chopped. Combine with grated cheddar.

In a separate bowl whisk the milk with eggs, cider vinegar and oil. Stir in almond flour, spices and baking soda. Stir until just combined. Add broccoli mix and stir to combine.

Form 12 patties/cookies and arrange onto baking sheet. Bake for 15 minutes, remove from the oven and re-form so they look like real cookies. Bake for 5 minutes more.

Turn oven to broil and broil the cookies for 5 minutes. Remove from the oven and place aside to cool. Serve after.

Low-carb corndogs

Enough to make: 4 pieces

Required time to prepare: 10 minutes

Ingredients:

-        4 chicken sausages, pre-cooked

-        2 tablespoons heavy cream

-        2 eggs

-        1 cup almond flour

-        1 teaspoon baking powder

-        ½ teaspoon salt

-        ½ teaspoon turmeric

Directions:

In a bowl mix together the almond flour and spices.

In a separate bowl whisk the eggs with heavy cream and baking powder. Fold the egg mixture into almond flour mix and stir until well combined.

Heat around 1 cup oil in large pan until reaches 400F, then Dip the pre-cooked sausages into almond flour mix and place into heated oil. Fry for 2 minutes per side or until golden.

Serve after.

Thyme onion rings

Enough to make: 2 rings

Required time to prepare: 30 minutes

Ingredients:

-       2 sweet onions, large

-       1 ½ cups almond flour

-       2 tablespoons thyme, fresh, chopped

-       ½ teaspoon salt

-       ½ teaspoon garlic powder

-       ½ teaspoon black pepper

-       2 eggs

Directions:

Preheat oven to 400F.

Wash and slice the onion into rings.

Combine the almond flour, thyme, salt, garlic powder and black pepper in a bowl. Whisk the eggs in separate bowl.

Dip each onion ring into egg mixture and dredge through flour mix. Arrange onion slices onto baking sheet.

Bake in preheated oven for 25 minutes, turning over halfway through. Serve while still hot.

Avocado fries

Enough to make: 2 pieces

Required time to prepare: 25 minutes

Ingredients:

- 2 avocados, sliced into ½-inch wedges

- ½ cup almond flour

- ¼ cup sunflower seeds, crushed

- 1 teaspoon salt

- ½ teaspoon onion powder

- 2 eggs, beaten

Directions:

Preheat oven to 450F and line baking sheet with parchment paper.

Whisk the eggs in shallow dish. In separate bowl combine the almond flour, sunflower seeds, and salt and onion powder.

Dip the avocado slices into egg mixture and coat with almond flour mix. Place onto baking sheet and bake for 20 minutes. Serve after.

Cauliflower bites

Enough to make: 4 bites

Required time to prepare: 15 minutes

Ingredients:

- 4 cups cauliflower florets
- 1 cup almond flour
- ¼ cup Parmesan, grated
- 2 eggs beaten
- 1 teaspoon cayenne
- 1 teaspoon garlic powder

Directions:

In a large bowl combine the almond flour, parmesan, cayenne pepper and garlic powder.

In a separate bowl whisk the eggs.

Dip the cauliflower florets into egg mixture and transfer in a bowl with almond flour mix. Toss to coat well.

Heat 2-inches oil in large skillet. Add cauliflower florets and cook for 2-3 minutes or until evenly golden. Place on paper towels to drain and serve.

Parmesan puffs

Enough to make: 12 puffs

Required time to prepare: 10 minutes

Ingredients:

- ½ cup oil, olive

- 4 egg whites

- ½ cup Parmesan, grated

- 1 teaspoon basil, dried

- 1 pinch salt

Directions:

Whip the egg whites with 1 pinch salt until soft peaks form.

Gently fold the parmesan and basil into the egg mixture.

Heat olive oil in large skillet and drop the egg white mix by spoon into hot oil.

Cook until browned on all sides, 5 minutes. Serve while still hot.

Beef jerky

Enough to make: 4 pieces

Required time to prepare: 2 hours + inactive time

Ingredients:

- 1lb. beef, grass-fed and lean

- ½ cup coconut amino

Directions:

Slightly freeze the meat so you can slice it nicely to 1/8-inch thick.

Place the beef slices in large zip-lock bag and add coconut amino; seal the bag and refrigerate the meat for 2 hours.

Preheat oven to 200F and line two baking sheets with aluminum foil and simply place wire rack onto baking sheet.

Place the marinated beef onto wire rack and bake or dehydrate for 2 hours.

Keep in airtight container.

Avocado snack

Enough to make: 1 piece

Required time to prepare: 5 minutes

Ingredients:

- 1 avocado cut in quarters

- 2 tablespoons sunflower seeds, crushed

Directions:

Peel avocado and cut in quarters.

Sprinkle with sunflower seeds and serve immediately.

Rosemary almonds

Enough to make: 2 pieces

Required time to prepare: 20 minutes

Ingredients:

- 2 cups almond, blanched

- 2 tablespoons fresh rosemary, chopped

- 1 teaspoon salt

- 2 tablespoons olive oil

- 1 teaspoon smoked paprika

Directions:

Hat large skillet over medium-high heat.

Coat with olive oil and heat up.

Add the almonds and stir so they do not burn up.

Reduce the heat to low and add salt, paprika and rosemary.

Cook for 2 minutes and place on kitchen towel.

Serve while still warm.

Zucchini fritters

Enough to make: 12 mini fritters

Required time to prepare: 10 minutes

Ingredients:

- 1 large zucchini, finely grated

- 1 ½ tablespoons grated parmesan cheese

- 1 egg, whisked

- Dash of chili flakes

- Fresh ground salt and pepper – just a pinch

- 2 tablespoons almond flour

Directions:

Place grated zucchinis in clean kitchen towel to remove excess liquid.

Place in a bowl and add remaining ingredients; stir well to combine.

Heat some oil in frying pan and add 1 tablespoon of zucchini mixture per fritter.

Cook fritters in batches, for 2 minutes per side or until golden.

Serve immediately with favorite sauce.

Bacon wrapped potatoes

Enough to make: 4 pieces

Required time to prepare: 30 minutes

Ingredients:

- 0.5 lb. Mini potatoes

- 7 oz. thick cut bacon

- Fresh ground pepper

- Fresh ground salt

- 1 teaspoon rosemary, chopped

- 1 tablespoon olive oil

- 1 teaspoon smoked paprika

Directions:

Wash, dry, and chop potatoes into 1-inch cubes.

Place the potatoes in medium size pot with salted boiling water.

Cook potatoes for 3-4 minutes.

Meanwhile, preheat oven to 420F and line baking tray with parchment paper.

Drain the potatoes and place in a bowl.

Season with salt and pepper. Add rosemary, smoked paprika, and olive oil.

Toss to combine, until potatoes are evenly coated.

Cut the bacon slices in halves and wrap around potatoes. Secure with toothpick.

Arrange onto baking sheet and bake for 15 minutes. Flip on other side and cook for 15 minutes more. Remove toothpicks before serving.

Avocado-tuna bites

Enough to make: 12 bites

Required time to prepare: 15 minutes

Ingredients:

- 10oz. can tuna, drained

- 1/3 cup almond flour

- 1 avocado, peeled, diced

- ¼ cup mayonnaise

- ¼ cup parmesan, grated

- ½ teaspoon salt

- ¼ teaspoon garlic powder

Directions:

In a bowl combine the tuna with mayonnaise, parmesan and spices.

Add the diced avocado and stir to combine.

Spread the almond flour in shallow dish.

From the 12 balls from the mixture and roll in almond flour

Heat 2-inch oil in large skillet; add prepared balls and cook until browned on all sides. Place on paper towel to drain, before serving.

Sweet snacks

Coconut bombs

Enough to make: 12 bombs

Required time to prepare: 10 minutes + inactive time

Ingredients:

- 4oz. flaked coconut

- ¼ cup coconut oil, melted

- ¼ teaspoon vanilla paste

- 20 drops Stevia

Directions:

Preheat oven to 350F and line baking sheet with parchment paper. Spread over coconut flakes and place in the oven.

Toast the flakes for 5-8 minutes until golden. Stir once to prevent burning.

Transfer in a blender and pulse until smooth.

Add the coconut oil, vanilla paste and Stevia. Stir to combine.

Divide between 12 mini paper cases and place in freezer for 30 minutes.

Once firm serve after.

Pecan bars

Enough to make: 12 bars

Required time to prepare: 30 minutes

Ingredients:

- 2 cups pecan halves, toasted, crushed

- ½ cup shredded coconut

- ½ cup coconut oil, melted

- ¼ teaspoon Stevia, liquid

- ½ cup golden flaxseeds meal

- 1 cup almond flour

- 2 tablespoons almond butter

Directions:

In a bowl combine the almond flour, flaxseeds meal and shredded coconut.

Add crushed pecans and stir again.

Add in remaining ingredients and mix well until you get a crumbly mixture.

Line 11x7-inch baking pan with parchment paper and place in the prepared mixture. Press to flatten and bake in preheated oven for 25 minutes at 350F.

Remove from the oven and allow being cool. Slice into bars and serve.

Peanut butter balls

Enough to make: 4 balls

Required time to prepare: 5 minutes + inactive time

Ingredients:

-	2 tablespoons heavy cream

-	4 tablespoons almond butter

-	2 tablespoon peanut butter, smooth

-	4 drops Stevia

-	1 ½ teaspoons powdered Erythritol

Directions:

In a bowl combine all ingredients. Mix until smooth.

Place in a freezer for 20 minutes. Form into balls and serve.

Strawberry snack

Enough to make: 4 pieces

Required time to prepare: 10 minutes + inactive time

Ingredients:

-        10 strawberries

-        ¼ cup almond flour

-        3oz. cream cheese

-        1 tablespoon powder Erythritol

-        ¼ teaspoon vanilla paste

Directions:

In a small bowl combine the cream cheese, vanilla and powder Erythritol.

Place the almond flour in a bowl.

Make a small hole in each strawberry and fill with cream cheese. Dip the strawberry tops in almond flour and refrigerate for 20 minutes before serving.

Pumpkin bombs

Enough to make: 2 bombs

Required time to prepare: 10 minutes + inactive time

Ingredients:

-        2 tablespoons coconut oil, melted

-        ½ stick butter, grass-fed, unsalted

-        ½ cup pumpkin puree

-        1 pinch nutmeg

-        ½ teaspoon allspice

-        1 pinch cinnamon

-        5 drops Stevia

Directions:

Heat coconut oil in microwave until hot; add butter and whip with fork until blended.

Keep whipping and stir in the pumpkin.

Add the spices and Stevia. Place the mixture into fridge until firm. Form balls from the mixture and serve.

Cinnamon crackers

Enough to make: 6

Required time to prepare: 30 minutes

Ingredients:

-       2 cups almond flour

-       1 egg

-       2 tablespoons coconut oil

-       2 teaspoons vanilla paste

-       ¼ cup Erythritol

-       2 teaspoons cinnamon

-       1 teaspoon baking soda

-       1 pinch salt

Directions:

Preheat oven to 300F.In a medium bowl combine the almond flour, Erythritol, cinnamon, baking soda and salt.

Whisk in the egg, coconut oil and vanilla paste. Mix until you get cohesive dough.

Place the dough onto large piece of parchment paper; cover with the second one and roll to ¼-inch thick. Pell off top piece of parchment paper and score the dough into desired shape. Transfer onto baking sheet and bake for 20-25 minutes.

Remove from the oven, allow being cool and breaking up along score marks. Bake for 15 minute more and serve after.

Mango fruit roll

Enough to make: 2 rolls

Required time to prepare: 10 minutes + inactive time

Ingredients:

- 4 mangoes, peeled and cubed

- 1 orange, juiced

- 2 tablespoons powder Erythritol

Directions:

Combine mango, orange juice and powder Erythritol in food processor; pulse until blended and smooth.

Line baking sheet with parchment paper and spread over mango puree in ¼-inch thick layer.

Dry the mango for 4-8 hours, depending on the thickness at 140F.

When the fruit leather is dry and not sticky to the touch, remove from the oven and peel from the paper; cut in long strips, 2-inches wide and roll before serving.

Apple chips

Enough to make: 6 chips

Required time to prepare: 2 hours

Ingredients:

- 2 apples, medium

- 2 tablespoons pumpkin pie spice

- 2 tablespoon powder Erythritol

Directions:

Preheat oven to 200C and line baking sheet with parchment paper.

Using a mandolin, slice the apples very thin. Place the apple slices onto baking sheet.

In a bowl combine the Erythritol and pumpkin pie spice; sprinkle all over apple slices.

Bake the apples for 2 hours and serve after.

Vanilla-macadamia fat bombs

Enough to make: 14 bites

Required time to prepare: 10 minutes + inactive time

Ingredients:

- 1 cup macadamia nuts

- 1 teaspoon vanilla paste

- ½ cup coconut oil, melted

- 10 drops Stevia

- 2 tablespoons powdered Erythritol

Directions:

In a food blender pulse the macadamia nuts until smooth.

In a bowl combine the coconut oil with Stevia, Erythritol and vanilla paste. Stir in processed macadamia nuts and stir to mix well. Spoon the mixture into silicone ice-cube tray and place in freezer for 30 minutes.

Pop the sweets from the silicone tray and serve.

Coconut bites

Enough to make: 4 bites

Required time to prepare: 50 minutes

Ingredients:

- 4 egg whites

- 1 tablespoon powdered Erythritol

- 3 cups desiccated coconut

- 1pinch salt

Directions:

Preheat oven to 350F and line baking sheet with parchment paper.

Whisk the egg whites with 1pinch salt until firm.

Gently stir in the powdered Erythritol and coconut.

Form the balls with hands and arrange onto baking sheet.

Bake the coconut balls for 45 minutes or until the balls crackle.

Remove and place aside to cool. Serve after.

Waffle sticks

Enough to make: 2 sticks

Required time to prepare: 15 minutes

Ingredients:

- 6 tablespoons almond flour

- 2 eggs

- ½ teaspoon vanilla paste

- 1 tablespoon Erythritol

- 1 teaspoon cinnamon

- ¼ teaspoon baking soda

Directions:

In a bowl combine the almond flour, Erythritol, ½ teaspoon cinnamon and baking soda.

Whisk in the eggs and vanilla paste.

Preheat waffle iron and pour over prepared batter. Cook the waffle for 3-4 minutes.

Cut waffle into sticks and sprinkle with remaining cinnamon. Serve after.

Apple and almond butter bites

Enough to make: 2 bites

Required time to prepare: 15 minutes

Ingredients:

- 1 apple, cored and sliced thinly

- 2 tablespoons almond butter

- 2 tablespoons crushed almonds

- 1 tablespoon pecans, crushed

Directions:

Spread the almond butter over apple slices.

Top each apple slice with crushed almonds and pecans.

Serve after.

Avocado-banana cacao cookies

Enough to make: 12 cookies

Required time to prepare: 25 minutes

Ingredients:

-       1 cup avocado, diced

-       ½ cup cacao powder, raw

-       1 tablespoon Erythritol

-       1 banana, sliced

-       1 egg

-       ½ teaspoon baking soda

Directions:

Preheat oven to 350F and line baking sheet with parchment paper.

Combine banana, Erythritol and avocado in a bowl.

Mix all until smooth and chunks free. Add the egg, cacao powder and baking soda. Continue mixing until everything is blended.

Drop spoonful of batter onto baking sheet and bake for 8-10 minutes. Place on wire rack to cool and serve after.

Conclusion

Much obliged to you again to download this book!

I trust this book could enable you to find some astounding Keto Recipes. The following stage is to get cooking!!!

As discussed, it is not necessary to suffer a lot to lose weight. Some small changes in your daily habits will make huge changes in your life

Also always remember that you are the one who can decide and take the actions.

Author Final words

Here we are, finally I just want to say you can do that as many people including myself had done before.

At long last, on the off chance that you delighted in this book, at that point I'd get a kick out of the chance to approach you for some help, would you be sufficiently benevolent to leave a survey for this book on Amazon? It'd be enormously refreshing!

Click here to leave a review for this book on Amazon

Thank you and good luck!

www.ingramcontent.com/pod-product-compliance
Lightning Source LLC
Chambersburg PA
CBHW051755250726
48659CB00001B/424